NURSING - ISSUES, PROBLEMS AND CHALLENGES

D1711343

WRITING FOR PUBLICATION

EASY-TO-FOLLOW TEMPLATE GUIDES FOR NURSES AND ALLIED HEALTH PROFESSIONALS

NURSING - ISSUES, PROBLEMS AND CHALLENGES

Additional books in this series can be found on Nova's website under the Series tab.

Additional e-books in this series can be found on Nova's website under the e-book tab.

NURSING - ISSUES, PROBLEMS AND CHALLENGES

WRITING FOR PUBLICATION

EASY-TO-FOLLOW TEMPLATE GUIDES FOR NURSES AND ALLIED HEALTH PROFESSIONALS

DARLENE SREDL, PH.D.

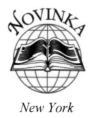

New York

Library of Congress Cataloging-in-Publication Data

ISBN: 978-1-63321-917-5

Library of Congress Control Number: 2014954523

Published by Nova Science Publishers, Inc. † New York

CONTENTS

PREFACE

WRITING FOR PUBLICATION: EASY- TO- FOLLOW TEMPLATE GUIDES
Darlene Sredl, Ph.D., R.N.

This book may well change the way you view writing. To many would-be authors writing is a laborious process in which the 'wheel' has to be reinvented over and over again. Not so! There are many forms of writing that utilize *templates* for directions. These act like recipes for a favorite dish, combining step-by-step instructions on how to cook or bake a traditional favorite.

If you attempted to cook beef stroganoff, for example, without using a recipe, you would have to go through the following steps: think about which ingredients might be necessary; shop for and buy the ingredients; assemble the appropriate equipment-pots, pans, mixing bowls; think about which steps in the cooking process should be completed first; think about which steps in the cooking process should be accomplished in a special chronological order, pre-heat the oven if required; combine certain ingredients-(for example, vermouth is an important flavor in this dish and it must be slowly boiled to reduce the amount by half as it evaporates the alcohol content). And on…and on… Do you see how much original thinking has gone into just trying to formulate a way to prepare this delicious dish?

If, on the other hand, you pulled out a recipe for beef stroganoff you would have at your fingertips a *TEMPLATE* instructing you on how to go about cooking this wonderful and flavorful dish-just follow the simple instructions, and VOILA! You have dinner! The template of a recipe has taken the guesswork and a lot of the painstaking thinking out of the preparation.

In a sense writing, using some of the basic templates shown herein, is a lot like using a recipe. Sure you still have to search the literature for content information, but assembling it into a cohesive article/essay/book/poem, or whatever has become 50% easier using the scaffolding structure of a *template*.

The first chapter is devoted to identifying writing types and styles; while the succeeding chapters cover sought after types of original writing pieces using graphic *templates*.

Title notwithstanding, this book is not primarily about writing. Any number of creative writing &/or English composition classes can teach you that. Rather, this book is about what you can do with your written words after you have finished writing---namely, how to publish them.

Decades of experience culminating in over 90 professional publications, countless public education articles, and five books have taught me that seeking a publisher; fitting your manuscript to the publisher's needs and audience, negotiating contract terms; and revising, editing, and formatting may well be a science unto itself. My experience has extended through publishing most types of writing. This experience with varied forms of writing also taught me that with many types of writing a template could be followed that can be modified and adapted to the various topic areas that you might be interested in developing.

These templates form the backbone of this book. Follow the template prompts and both your writing and your efforts toward publication will become much easier- and hopefully- more successful!

Dr. Darlene Sredl, Ph.D., R.N.
Teaching Professor of Nursing
College of Nursing
University of Missouri @ St. Louis
Chesterfield, MO, 63005
Tel: 636-391-9277
E-mail: Sredld@umsl.edu

Chapter 1

EXPOSITORY VERSUS NARRATIVE WRITING

TIPS YOU SHOULD KNOW

This chapter explores some of the more common types and styles of writing. It is important to discuss the basic tenets of each because you will see examples of them (with *templates*) in the succeeding chapters.

The word 'expository' really means that it offers an explanation or provides some form of information. Hopefully all printed material does this to some extent. The last thing publishers want to see is a rehash of old information. They know readers pick up their publication to learn something new. In this economy printed paper journals and books cost a lot in ink, paper, and people-power. These costs must be bourne by subscribers wishing to learn something new; new information or techniques. Advertisers, who also bear some of the publishing costs of the published entity, only want to put their money in publications that they know have wide reader appeal.

So…you, the writer, have to provide the new content. That is **writer tip #1**. You can provide new content in either expository or narrative form. Let's explore each.

EXPOSITORY

EXPOSITORY-Descriptive

Descriptive writing relies on the author providing a lot of background information to 'set the stage' so to speak for the application of the new factual information. We see this type of writing in historical documents and in user manuals as well as in some fiction.

EXPOSITORY-Explanatory

Explanatory writing requires the author to root out causes for the occurrence of some result. This form of writing relies heavily on theory. It may be the form of writing you see in clinical research articles.

EXPOSITORY-Illustrative

Illustrative writing relies on supplements to the narrative such as might be seen with the inclusion of photographs, art, cartoons, and pictures of interest capturing the content of the essay.

EXPOSITORY-Analytical

Analytical writing conjures new information by identifying patterns or categories of activity related to the assimilation of content provided in the essay. In the 1980's Howard Gardner posed his Theory of Multiple Intelligences. This theory postulated that human beings are capable of learning through eight (later expanded to ten) modes of accepting and assimilating information. The theory in total is very enlightening but for the purposes of our writing we shall only discuss one part of his theory here, that of-identifying patterns in nature.

All health professions, and other professions as well, rely on observations of phenomena that cluster around patterns. In nature we see how all the leaves of a particular species of tree or flower, for example, have the same look. If you plant a seed from that tree or flower you can be relatively sure the sprouting growth will look like the biological that the seed came from.

In the health sciences, professionals look for clusters of *symptoms* that occur with regularity in certain diseases. The identification of those symptoms help medical professionals identify the underlying disease process and aid in diagnosis.

Mathematicians rely on theorems developed through numerical patterns. Statisticians rely on clustered numbers we call 'central tendencies' to help explain cause and effect observations in clinical research studies.

ARGUMENTATIVE

Argumentative writing is mainly utilized within the profession of law, but also within any writing context in which a strong position must be either supported or debunked. It also relies heavily on personal opinion in interpreting the factual data. Debate covering both sides of an issue is expected with heavier reliance on the author's own position.

DEFINING-Evaluative

Evaluative writing requires the author to pass judgment or take sides in a philosophical essay. Competing definitions of the content are often evident and must be sorted out. This type of writing is seen in the technique of concept analysis. Concept analysis utilizes a combination of expository AND narrative writing in attempting to clearly define a word or commonly used phrase.

DEFINING-Interpretive

Interpretive defining writing allows the author freedom in offering his/her own personal opinion in place of other, more established, interpretations of some selected information. This can be found in cartoons or text covering political satire. It is also the technique of choice in rebutting the opinions of other published authors. [1]

Writer tip #2-Many essays involve combinations of two or more of the above techniques such as are found in this text.

NARRATIVE WRITING

Narrative Writing Fiction

Narrative writing is fun; especially if it is fiction! You can let your imagination run amuck and be totally amazed and, sometimes, delighted at how your characters come to life. There is no template for narrative writing, but also no hard and fast rules. Introduce, then, grow your characters personality-wise and situationally-wise.

One of the professional forums discussed in a later chapter is Concept Analysis. This form of writing does utilize a template and also requires fictional narrative writing as a way of developing the case studies required as part of the template. See CONCEPT ANALYSIS (sp) in Chapter 4 for more details.

The Role of a Literary Agent

Magazines and e-zines have a voracious appetite for quality fiction. This is also a very competitive market and may require the services of a literary agent to get your work reviewed especially if you do not have a publication dossier yet built up. The literary agent who agrees to represent your work may offer services to review, critique and enhance your written work but be aware that these services are often pricey.

The literary agent will also submit your finalized work to a journal. When your work is accepted, the literary agent will bill you a contracted agreed upon amount-usually a percentage of the honorarium paid by the journal.

Writer's Tip #3 Have fun with your fiction writing!

References

[1]   Mariconda, B., *Step-by-Step Strategies for Teaching Expository Writing*. 2001, New York: Scholastic Professional Books.

Chapter 2

THE IMPORTANCE OF CREATIVITY AND INITIATIVE

You can earn extra income writing for professional publication …in your spare time. Now, having said this, I wish to clarify-This is NOT a book about 'writing'. This is also NOT a book about 'English'. You can take those courses in school-excel in them, and still not be able to produce a publishable document. THIS IS A BOOK ABOUT *PUBLISHING*-fulfilling your dreams, and seeing your work in print for everyone else to see too. It is written in an easily understandable conversation style. Why do I think you can do this? Because your daily work in healthcare provides between 8-12 hours per shift of exciting experiences. If you keep a diary of situations, emotions, and practice setting descriptions you have all the rich background material to use as a setting for your material.

Creative thoughts can also help you win contests and bring in prizes and cash. Many, many years ago I learned of an acquaintance who won $25,000 in a contest. Contestants were asked to explain (in 25 words or less) why a particular brand of margarine was better than butter. I am sure most of the entries contained delicious and descriptive adjectives why the margarine was better, but consider this. Those marketing folks could wield a dictionary AND a thesaurus as well as anybody. The reason they were willing to put up the big bucks was to find something *different*-a *different angle*- a *new way* to promote and advertise the product-and…descriptive adjectives were not going to do that. My acquaintance won with these 3 words: "LESS SATURATED FAT". It changed the way fats and oils were thought of from that point on-AND led to healthier food for all of us.

Perhaps you are artistic? You can put your artistic creativity to use in drawing and captioning funny situations.

Your talent and skill as a photographer can also be put to use in helping to sell your writing. Photos that cover the article content usually bring extra honoraria when coupled with the submitted article.

CREATIVITY

Ah, how to get started. First forget the common myth that 'the muse of inspiration has to come first'. You will waste years waiting for that muse to show up-and what if she decides not to show up at all? No, you must take responsibility for coaxing that muse to show up and help you EVERY DAY. How, you ask? If you have ever turned in an assignment in school you already know how. You didn't wait for any imaginary 'muse' to show up. The assignments were listed on the course syllabus along with a date for their expected completion. You did the assignment on or before the date and turned in either a paper copy or an email attachment on that date. You FORCED the muse to help you! Of course it also took considerable reading, sitting through many lectures, sleeping when you could, AND finally sitting at your blank Word document and typing in some thoughts on the subject. The time you spent reading, sitting through lectures & sleeping was not wasted time-it was important for creativity to gestate and incubate into thoughts toward the topic you would eventually write about.

Nurturing the aptitude for creativity is perhaps the best example of what you can do to become a published author. Becoming a writer who is a published author is not just a happenstance occurrence. First, one must sincerely believe that others 'out there' want to know what is in your mind & on your mind. Have you had some exciting experiences? Do you have a challenging job that stimulates problem-solving on a regular basis? Have you taken, or are you planning on taking a trip to an exotic location? All of these scenarios are ripe for writing about-but not necessarily ripe for being published. That will take extra skill; BUT with the right coaching supplied by this book it should put your work under the noses of agreeable Editors-in-Chief who want to publish what you have written.

During your creative incubation stage, try to connect the dots of facts that might seem related although strikingly different. You may find that you are your most creative at night. Keep a pen and paper handy under your bed so that if you wake up at night with just the right phrase in mind you can quickly jot it down, then return to blissful sleep and hopefully more creative thoughts. If you think you don't have to do this & that you will surely remember the wording the next morning you are deceiving yourself. You won't remember it! So, write it down as you think of it. In fact keep a pen and small notebook on your person at all times because you never know when inspiration may strike.

You may be thinking-"I am not creative". If you think that (or worse, say it out loud) you are shooting yourself in the foot and all your publishing dreams with it. Around the turn of the twentieth century Napoleon Hill interviewed famous people of his day seeking to find out if there were any personality traits that successful people had that possibly other, not so successful, people did not have as much of. Creativity was one of the fifteen personality traits that he discovered in interviewing the successful people of his time (Henry Ford, the Wright brothers, Mark Twain). After six years of working as a nurse in the Neonatal Intensive Care Unit (NICU) I can personally attest to the fact that there was never a baby born who had creativity. Creativity is an ACQUIRED TRAIT. *You* can acquire that trait too. Try to think of ways of saying something in a unique way that also imparts, or alludes to other information.

For example, consider this statement: The men knew that this was a house of prostitution. (Factual but no promise)

Then consider this, more creatively written, statement: The men were excited at the thought of opportunities that lay, apparently, behind every door. (Plenty of promise)

Or, consider these examples: The children dragged many toys outside to play with. (DULL)

Then, consider this more creatively descriptive statement by Erma Bombeck:

The children wearied of dragging Daddy's power tools into the sandbox because they didn't work. (SURPRISING!).

From these examples one can see how the initial statement can be pushed, pulled, and/or bullied into becoming a more creative sentence just by changing a few words or by changing the intent. Also, remember the theory that states, "anything that surprises or delights is more likely to be remembered."

Taking INITIATIVE

No matter what it is that you are thinking of writing about, the matter will remain just a thought until you put those thoughts on paper (or, computer) and make some CONNECTION with an editor who just might want to publish your thoughts. Many people grow into old age saying 'I could write a book…" but they never do. The marvelous and insight-filled experiences they have been blessed with die with them. As a matter of fact-this very thing was spoken in my class one day and I found it so profound that I wrote a book based upon the wisdom of it.

The student said, "It's a shame that when doctors die their wonderful bedside manner dies with them because they never confided in anyone to teach them the secrets of successfully dealing with patients."

When I pondered this wisdom, I realized that nurses do the same thing & quite possibly other medical and scientific disciplines did it also. This, coupled with the fact that I teach Management and Leadership for Nurses, led me to propose a book to Nova Science Publishers (the publishers of this book too). My thought, based on my student's comment, was to solicit 'stories' from nurses and others in management positions in which the situation they were involved in looked very dour but, because of something they did or said, they turned the situation around and it ended on a positive note. My thought was that although fledgling nurse managers would probably never encounter the exact same problem, they might encounter something similar and could apply management principles to help guide them through the dour situation. The work evolved as time went by. I sent letters to top nursing managers and actively solicited stories of advice from others whom I knew personally had turned lemons into lemonade. Other stories I wrote myself that exemplified a few of the categories I wanted to include. As I read the stories that I had accepted, I saw that I could define the management/leadership principle(s) that were in play in each story. I also decided to identify both a nursing and a non-nursing theory that affected the positive outcome of each story. Finally I limited most of my references to the last ten years to make my information more recent and 'evidence-based'. [1]

Another example of this concept of "I could write a book, but…"involves the wildly popular book, *Heaven is For Real.* This book is about a middle class, American family with a young son who barely survived a devastating illness. That part of the story is very engaging just by itself; however, after his son recovers, the son drops little tidbits of what it was like being in heaven. A three year old would never come up with a story all at once. So, the family received little presents (sometimes wrapped in an enigma like when Colton said "Dad, Jesus has markers!") from time to time. Since Colton's father was a minister he did tell Colton's story from the pulpit. Supportive believers told him, "you should write a book". He didn't know where to begin. BUT...he finally did contact a publisher who wanted to publish the book if it got written and provided him with a helpful 'ghost-writer' (Lynn Vincent) [2] to help him write it. More about ghost-writers later- but know that they are out there and can be very helpful.

The theorist Napoleon Hill captured fifteen personality characteristics of successful people identified 'taking initiative' as one of them. [3] After all, if you don't take initiative and move forward in the direction of that initiative, NOTHING WILL HAPPEN.

KEEPING A DIARY

One of the most important things a 'would-be' writer can do is to develop the habit of keeping a diary. Whenever you are about to tackle a new project, take a course, go on an exotic vacation or whatever is the start of something important to you, the habit of writing in your diary on a daily basis will become an invaluable source of background material. You may or may not choose to use parts of it at a later date. Your diary notes should include a brief synopsis of the day's (or night's) activities, some unusual conversations, your emotions and how you felt about what was going on, etc.

I did this when I decided to become a pilot. As the flying lessons progressed, I wrote about what I learned & what I simply could not seem to grasp; my frustrations; pithy conversations involving me and those around me; and spectacular incidents- like the time I felt unusually incompetent praying for an answer whether or not I should continue this financially and emotionally draining project-when suddenly I flew through a vertical rainbow! The prism of cockpit glass shattered the colors making it look like someone had tossed a handful of sparkling jewels - garnets, amethysts, citrines, blue topazes & emeralds that floated around the cockpit for a few seconds. That brief encounter was all I needed. I had my answer. Continue despite all the obstacles and barriers. I am so glad I did. The diary of emotional expenditures endured during my pilot training provided the background material for my first book of fiction, *Pilot Quest* [4]. The knowledge gained through my flight training, coupled with my nursing knowledge provided a seemingly unlimited source of content for other book chapters, and journal articles that I was invited to write.

Todd Burpo, author of *Heaven is for Real*, also found journaling the day's events an important way to later remember his son, Colter's, memories of being in heaven during his out-of-body health crisis experience.

Developing the habit of writing in your diary at the end of every day will provide you with much fodder for your imagination when the time comes to put everything together into a book. Like any other habit we choose to develop, it requires a certain amount of repetition in order to make a function become a habit. Some have said it takes three weeks to either make or break a habit. Why do you want to make keeping a diary a habit? Because when you are writing that book it will provide valuable background information to 'flesh out' your topic; whereas not having enough background material may present the biggest stumbling block to developing your main topic

TITLE- A COMPELLING INTRODUCTION THAT LEAVES READERS WANTING MORE

One of the quickest ways to get an editor's attention is by providing an interesting title for your work. Remember, a provocative title will help the editors sell journals. Sure the content is important but if the title catches their attention, it will most probably catch their audience's interest too and result in an article acceptance for you. I learned this in the most surprising way. My article on "Cervical cancer" had been accepted by a leading LPN nursing journal. I was anxious to see it in print. Then came the publication and my professional article under the ignominious title, "Is there sex after...?" I was both astounded and embarrassed-**but**...I did learn the value of a provocative title. Now, when I say 'provocative' I don't necessarily mean it has to have sexual overtones. Provocative can actually mean a play on words relating to what is going on in the world. Here are two cases as examples.

When the US teetered on war concerned with 'Weapons of Mass Destruction' that might possibly be hidden in Iraq, I was researching lung transplantation. My article with a very mundane title did not get accepted by the professional journals that I wanted to accept it. Finally I changed the title to:

Words of Mass Persuasion: A Literature Review of Cognitive Behavioural Therapy (CBT) and Message-Based Persuasion Systems (MBPS) Use in Adolescent Transplant Depression. [5]

I am sure that the alliterative phrase, 'Words of Mass Persuasion' sounded enough like ' Weapons of Mass Destruction' to make the editors take a second look-and, decide to accept my article for it's timeliness.

Another research study, examining 'Evidence-Base Nursing Process (EBNP) comprehension among Chief Nurse Executives (CNE)' got nowhere with that bland title. When I changed the title to:

Healthcare in crisis! Can nurse executives' beliefs about, and implementation of, Evidence-Based Practice (EBP) be key solutions in healthcare reform? It was accepted by the first journal I sent it to [6]. This occurred around the time of the great Presidential push toward ratification of the law now known as the Affordable Care Act, commonly referred to as 'Obamacare'. The exaggerated 'crisis' of skyrocketing health care costs provided a better title proposing EBNP as a solution for the 'crisis'.

GHOST WRITERS

Ghost writers, as mentioned earlier in this chapter, are professional writers who agree to help an author write a book. This verbal agreement is also accompanied by a contract, a fee, a Byline next to the original author's, and possibly a percentage of royalties. There is a marked benefit to the original author in that the ghost writer has a writing style already developed that can be applied to the original author's content material. There is a marked benefit to the ghost writer in that he/she can write without having to forage up content-it is being spoon-fed to him/her. The writing process can proceed by many different ways depending upon the original author's and the ghost writer's preference. Sometimes the original author will actually write short vignettes of the story with the ghost writer embellishing, polishing, and finishing it up. Other authors prefer to either speak directly to the ghost writer or speak into a recorder that the ghost writer can pick up from time to time and transcribe. I have been asked by colleagues to assist with the writing of their research studies-another form of ghost writing.

FICTION SUPPORTED BY FACT

A. Fiction Supported by Fact

Earlier we discussed the importance of keeping a daily diary or journal in which one could log entries of what was done, or seen that day; what emotions were felt, what was said, what could have been improved upon, etc. The importance of writing in this journal at the start of a new venture, or an unusual or exotic trip, or any kind of novel undertaking cannot be overemphasized. The material can be reviewed at a later date to provide accurate background material for a fictional topic you may wish to write about. Guaranteed you will not be able to remember these fine nuances without the prompts offered by your journal entries.

When I decided to become a pilot, I also realized that it might lead to rich material that could be used later, or I might fail and not be able to use the material at all. That was OK, although I did not wish to fail. So, by journaling each day's flight activities I was able to capture my frustrations with battling the crosswinds, coping with mysogenistic established pilots whose culture did not include female pilots, and the stressors of each new flight environment I found myself having to conquer.

When I decide to write a fictional book about a nurse executive who wanted to pursue a lifelong goal, I was able to use the journal and put the chronological experiences together to form a cohesive background for the story. So, the fiction is the imaginary family structure I created and the facts are found in the sequences of gaining more and more expertise in flying. [7]

No matter what type of 'story' you wish to create (romance, adventure, travel, science fiction), if you want to write fiction, your habit of keeping a diary will come to your aid in writing that story. Popular thought says that you 'should write about what you know'. It is good advice. Many times, however, that is the exact thing that stymies the author in starting to write. The author may have a good idea of an engaging topic but think that the background that he knows is too mundane to write about. And...he may be right. Why not transplant the story to another location that he also knows-maybe drawn from his vacation in Barbados? Reviewing the hastily scribbled pages of his diary he will BE AMAZED at the wealth of usable information he finds just waiting to be inserted into the action.

An outline is also an indispensable way to begin your story but don't be surprised if that supporting skeleton disintegrates shortly into the action as the characters come to life and make decisions on their own. This is why it is so exciting to write fiction! When I wrote *Pilot Quest* [7] I originally intended it to be semi-autobiographical. I utilized my flight school diary to insert usual and unusual flying sequences, for background action and to maintain compelling reader interest. *However…*very shortly into the writing process my characters went AWOL, deserting the original outline. They took on their own distinctive personalities and did what THEY wanted to-not what I had prescribed in my outline. So, it became a work of fiction even though I used my student flight experiences as background material to flesh out the story line.

SCREEN WRITING

Have you ever noticed how many books, TV shows, and Broadway plays follow a common format that has been used successfully time and time again to develop the central theme? Among Broadway plays, *A Chorus Line*, and *Rent*, and the movies *Airplane* and *Airport* have all their characters housed in one place. In *A Chorus Line* the characters reveal themselves by dialogue during their backstage rehearsals.

In the play, Rent, the venue is an apartment building. The characters are the occupants of the building and their stories unfoldin a similar manner. The main thread of conflict holding them together was the potential that the building might be condemned and they would all have to find new living quarters. In *Rent* we get to peek into each apartment and see the characters as their personalities and goals are revealed in their domicile setting within one apartment building.

In the movie *Airplane*, the plot revolves around individual concerns of selected passengers on one airplane on one ill-fated flight. In *Airport* the main characters are the administrative team grappling with potentially dangerous developments among their aircraft. Are you beginning to see the similarities among all these different writing venues? A more recent addition to use of this writing template is the movie *The Beautiful and Exotic Marigold Hotel*. In this movie the audience is introduced to people facing financial difficulties so profound that they decide to move to India and live in the Marigold Hotel.

Use of this template for writing allows the authors to develop characters each with special problems in special circumstances that also contribute to the story tension. Yes, I said 'tension'. Without a certain amount of tension in the script the audience would soon get bored and give up on the story. Who wants to continue reading or viewing a boring story? No one! So, character development and plot tension development must proceed together to make the audience want to continue reading toward a resolved (and believable) conclusion. To do this, the characters in these singular settings are introduced one by one along with the unique set of troubling circumstances they find themselves in as well as the overarching problem that menaces their survival. In *A Chorus Line* the menacing problem that gradually unfolds concerns one aspiring but aging dancer's desire for a job in the new show despite a romantic but estranged history with the show's choreographer.

Healthcare professionals can easily see how their experiences during the course of their work can be applied to this template. Using the venue of the hospital, a few patients and their family situations can be developed along with a few key medical personnel caring for them. The main thread of focus can be some situation that may potentially destroy the hospital- possibly a tornado storm, or fire, etc. The main caution of using these situations is to keep characters anonymous so that the story line cannot be easily traced to anyone. It is also a good idea to issue a disclaimer on the copyright page that the characters within the book are fictional.

There have been many Broadway plays and movies produced in the last few years that have followed a successful template time and time again. The Broadway plays, A Chorus Line and Rent used the template of a common location with characters vying for recognition. As each of the main characters were introduced, their personalities developed and their relationship to one another evolved. In A Chorus Line the venue was backstage chorus selection and rehearsal for a new play about to open on Broadway. Each aspiring dancer told how important getting this job was to her and a little bit about their background. As the story developed one dancer's story evolved to reveal a former relationship with the director that might conflict with and hinder her aspirations for being selected for this job. All needing a job was the main thread of the story.

In a similar manner, the movies Airplane and Airport, were filmed in an airplane and an airport respectively. By now you get the picture, each passenger in the airplane or each administrative person working in the airport was wthin the cast of characters whose special circumstances to the situation were explored while the main thread of conflict involved either the potential for the plane to crash or some terrorist activity affecting the airport.

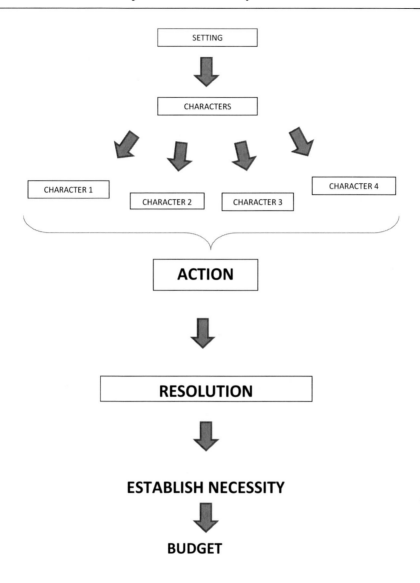

Figure/Template 1-1. Screen writing.

Using This Template

Health care workers have a wealth of characters, venues and conflict situations with which to use this template to develop a script. The venue might be a cardiac unit in a hospital. The characters could be two or three patients &

their families concerned about their illness (or, upcoming surgery); and possibly two or three healthcare workers with issues of their own that might adversely affect the patients.

Cartoons

A Nurse or Allied Health professional's perspective on situations occurring in the healthcare arena can be very funny indeed. One need not have a degree in graphic art or Photoshop to use a marking pen to sketch out a few humorous ideas. For example:

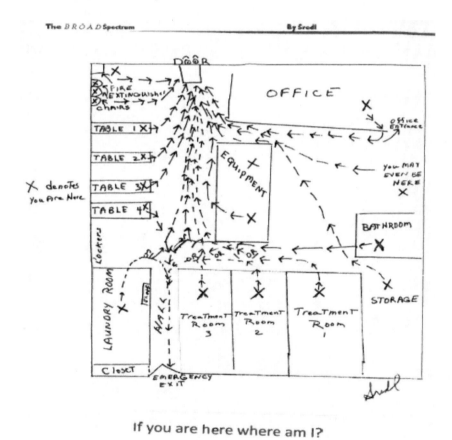

Figure/Template 1-2. "If you are here, where am I"?

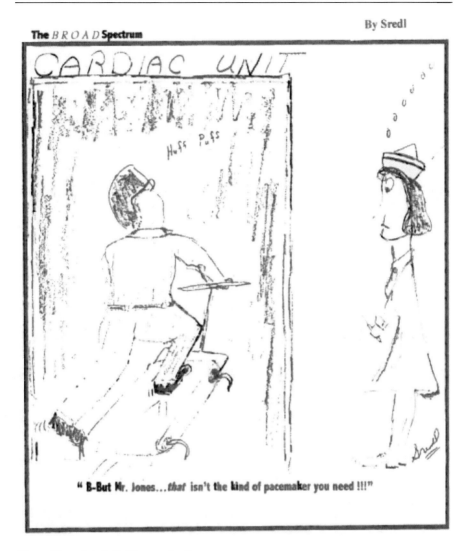

Figure/Template 1-3. "Pacemaker".

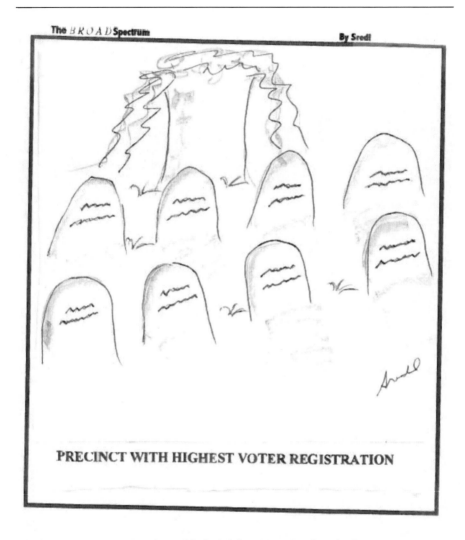

Figure/Template 1-4. "Precinct with the Highest Voter Registration".

REFERENCES

[1]   Sredl, D.E., *Evidence-Based Leadership Success Strategies for Nurse Administrators, Advance Practice Nurses (APN), and Doctors of Nursing Practice* (DNP). 2012, Hauppauge, N.Y.: Nova Science Publishers.
[2]   Burpo, T., *Heaven is for Real.* 2010, Nashville: W. Publishing Group.
[3]   Hill, N., *Law of Success.* Chicago: Success Unlimited Publishers.

[4]   Sredl, D., *Pilot Quest.* 2005, Boston: PublishAmerica.

[5]   Sredl, D., Words of Mass Persuasion: A Literature Review of CognitiveBehavioural Therapy (CBT) and Message-Based Persuasion Systems (MBPS) Use in Adolescent Transplant Depression. *Transplant Nurses Journal* (Australia), 2005. 14(1): p. 8-16.

[6]   Sredl, D., Jenkins, R., Hsiang, K.,Ding, C., Durham, J., Healthcare in crisis! Can nurse executives' beliefs about, and implementation of, Evidence-Based Practice (EBP) be key solutions in healthcare reform? *The Journal of Teaching and Learning in Nursing,* 2011. 6: p. 73-79.

[7]   Sredl, D., *Pilot Quest.* 2007, Frederick, MD: PublishAmerica.

Chapter 3

TYPES OF IDEAS WORTH SUBMITTING TO A PUBLISHER

PERSONAL OPINION

As a credentialed professional, YOUR ideas are considered 'pedigreed'. That means that the alphabet soup of letters following your name in the article's byline indicates to the reader that the opinions expressed in the article are not merely empty inflated conjecture- no, they are based upon a body of specific knowledge to which you are adding your personal thoughts. One of my relatives had a background in sheet metal. He later took a position in a technical college to teach the mechanics of sheet metal work to students aspiring to enter the trade. He was appalled at the lack of resources available to help the students. So…he set about writing a book about the basics of sheet metallurgy using his extensive training and experience as a seasoned professional. One book led to another…then another…six books in all! Of course he used those books as required texts in his courses (thereby bolstering his meager teacher's salary)-but more importantly, those books were also used in technical colleges throughout the United States due to the "books in print" listing by the Library of Congress. This listing can be consulted by anyone looking to find the latest book of information on a given topic. Needless to say, he retired a millionaire!

LETTERS TO THE EDITOR

There may be times when you have an idea that is still in the gestational stage-not quite well established enough to develop an entire article around it-but still significant enough that you want to get the idea 'out there' in the court of public opinion to get noticed. In that case you can write a 'Letter to the Editor' of a journal that deals with the subject matter you wish to write about. Letters that ultimately get published concern some new factual information or a synthesis of observations from specialists. For example, one of my nursing students who worked on a cardiology floor was concerned about the number of patients that she observed having depressive symptoms after receiving the diagnosis that they were in 'heart failure'. She deduced that the phrase in itself was formidable and set in motion the depressive symptoms that she observed-sad affect, loss of zest for living, appetite and sleep disturbances, crying, etc. Her contention was to change the wording on the diagnosis of 'heart failure' to something less scary to patients. Her letter was published by the Journal of Cardiac Nursing and the subject was later taken up at a discussion during the Cardiology Physicians Conference. One never knows how far-reaching the effects of your thinking will be.

OTHER AUTHOR POSITION REFUTATION

Another, relatively little used area of writing, involves taking issue with something another author has written. Many professional journals actively seek articles by top authorities in their field. These articles are often personal opinion articles based upon the author's experience. A clever author can poke holes in the published author's argument and, if presented in a logical yet respectful manner, backed up by factual data, may be very publishable indeed. Editors feel they have a duty to present both sides of an argument so this type of writing finds editorial approval more times than naught.

I took exception with an article in the prestigious *Journal of Advanced Nursing*, wrote a refutation within 2 months of the original article's publication date and it was accepted four months later with no request for revision. In cases like this, the editor will reference the article under contention but it remains the reader's prerogative to look up and read the original article before reading the refutation. How often this is actually done, I have no idea;

but the technique is a relatively easy template to follow if one needs/wants a quick publication under his/her belt.

Sredl, D. (2001). Response to 'The idea of nursing science' by S.D. Edwards (1999). Journal of Advanced Nursing 35(3), 386-387. [1]

NEW TWIST ON AN OLD IDEA

One thing editors absolutely HATE is receiving an over-the-transom (translation- a submitted article that was not expected or requested) article that was only a rehash of other articles. Newsprint, paper, postage and even Web space is too costly to use unless the subject matter is NEW, FRESH and/or based upon empirical research. New findings from an empirical study are more likely to get published IF those findings are positive. Findings that are not substantiated are less likely to find editorial approval unless it is a slow month editorially speaking. [2]

This is not to say however that you HAVE to set up an entirely new clinical trial, and go through the rigors of a 1 to 2 year research study in order to qualify for publication under this premise. IF you can use your creativity to restructure existing information from a NEW ANGLE, it also can be publishable. Here is an example of that:

In the 1990s SARS appeared on the healthcare scene globally. There was a lot of information about SARS but it was all written by physicians based on information put out by the Center for Disease Control (CDC). I could not find a single article on SARS written by a nurse. I definitely wanted to be the first nurse to author an article on SARS. But...what to write? I just said that editors were not interested in a rehash of old information, so what could I write about?

Then an idea dawned. My creativity *and* professional education kicked in. Since SARS was a respiratory disease, and I was a nurse trained in the symptomatology of respiratory (as well as other) diseases, why not develop a table of SARS symptoms and compare them to symptoms of other respiratory diseases, like pneumonia, RSV (respiratory syncytial virus), influenza, emphysema, chronic obstructive pulmonary disease (COPD), and the like? The table and accompanying narrative was a huge success and snapped up by a well-respected nursing journal. [3]

Sredl, D. (2003). Sars: Here today and gone tomorrow? *Nursing Made Incredibly* Easy 1(2), 28-36 *CE credit.*

At other times editors may be looking for topics loosely related to each other on a special theme. On one occasion I wrote an article entitled "New therapies for decubitus ulcer (bedsore) management" that was accepted by a popular nursing journal. The journal, however, took too long in my estimation, to publish the article. I wrote back rescinding my permission to publish stating that so much time had passed since article acceptance that the therapies were no longer 'new'. The editor apologized and asked if I would accept a 'kill fee' of $200 for their complacency. I accepted. A few months after that I was surprised to see a big article about bedsores complete with a glossy centerfold four color picture of a particularly gruesome stage four decubitus ulcer example. There, among seven other small-font articles about bedsores *was my article*! I had accepted the kill fee so the article was theirs to do with as they pleased-they bought and paid for it. My guess is that they had done the same for the other authors and then had so many related articles they decided to make a composite article featuring all of them. Certainly a clever solution on their part. [4]

Sredl, D. (1986)."More pressure sore treatments and why they're used. *RN(1)*, 39.

PERSONAL EXPERIENCE

One of the more satisfying ways to get published, and perhaps the easiest to write, is YOUR personal experience. You don't have to have a Ph.D. or a DNP to do this. Every time you go to work your shift assignment is full of potential stories to write about. Did you care for a patient with an unusual disease process? If so you have the opportunity within the body of the article that you write to educate others about this unusual disease process. Did you form a special relationship with your patient or her family, or, perhaps with another co-worker as a result of working together on some committee or other project? Did something humorous happen at work; or, something extremely sad? Did you help someone achieve a goal? ALL of these types of situations are fodder for an article that editors and journal readers will find interesting.

One of my nursing students told of three consecutive clinical days in which on the first day he cared for a pre-transplant patient; on the second he was allowed to observe the transplant surgery; and on the third he cared for the post-transplant patient. I encouraged him to write about these phenomenal serial clinical experiences. He did and his article was accepted in *Interim, The Journal of Student Nursing*.

In my own life, I went through a creative drought during a long health crisis. My femur broke after a hip replacement and, refusing to heal, had the audacity to re-break three more times. My bones were technically classified as a non-union. I did not know if I could or would ever be able to hold a nursing position again. Then, something happened during my last hospital stay and it turned my emotional equilibrium around 360 degrees. When I decided to write about it, the article practically wrote itself. All the words came spilling out as fast as I could type them. I submitted the article, "Helping from my Hospital Bed," with very little rewriting and it was accepted by the first journal I sent it to. [5]

One of my assignments working on a Pediatric cardio-thoracic unit was to prepare an 8 year old boy for a lung transplant. He and his family arrived and he walked in looking like the picture of health. He was not even carrying an oxygen tote. I wondered how a new lung could help him when he did not seem to be in any distress? To make a long story short, he died on the operating table-as I watched! A fog of depression settled in over me that lasted six months. I questioned why I still worked on that unit. I questioned the outcomes of the transplant process itself.

Then one day while working on the unit, the intercom blared—"Mrs. Sredl come to the nurse's station!" There stood a mother and one of my former lung transplant patients. They had come from out-of-town for one of his regular post-transplant biopsies. Then, decided to come up and see if I was working that day. She told me how changed for the better her son had been; playing football with neighbor kids and not struggling to draw every breath as he had before. She told me what a good nurse I was and how they appreciated my care for their son. The incident brought me full circle in dealing with my former questions and doubts. The fog lifted that day and "Danny" was the result. [6]

PUBLISHING ETHICS

(Now, a word of caution here- publishing ethics requires that you submit an article *to only one journal at a time*. One has to wait till the editor either makes a decision to publish or notifies you that the article has been sent out to referees for an opinion-which takes a little longer. If after that time the decision is 'no' you may then begin the process all over again by submitting to another journal).

INTERVIEW

As we move through various positions and job categories in healthcare inevitably we come across strong leaders or managers whom we would like to emulate. These people may, in fact, be movers and shakers within their profession. Conducting a formal interview and writing the resultant interview for possible publication is an excellent way to get published. In addition to furthering identification of your own byline, this type of article calls attention to the interviewee's accomplishments and validates their contribution to their profession.

Preparations for the interview start with a formal request to the person you wish to interview. This is best done in person or by phone call. The person can then ask questions of what you are trying to accomplish within the interview; what will be the focus of the resultant article you propose to write; and which journal you are planning to submit to. During the course of this preliminary contact you will also have the opportunity to request an emailed copy of the interviewee's curriculum Vitae (CV) and permission to record the interview for clarification. You should also have at least a rudimentary idea of what you want to focus on and tell the person you wish to interview that you will email him/her a list of questions so that he/she will have some time to gather behavioral responses (exemplary stories) to your questions. This eliminates most of the hemming and hawing to fill in quiet voids as the interviewee thinks of responses to your questions ahead of time. Advise your subject that the interview will probably take between 1 and one-and-a-half hours so they will know how much time to block out in their daily schedule.

If you have an idea of what will be your main focus, you could also use this opportunity to contact the Editor-in-Chief of a professional journal that focuses on topics of the sort you plan to write about to see if they would be interested in reviewing your proposed article once it is completed. Be sure to examine the journal's Website for details regarding author guidelines so that you may format your article according to that journal's requirements.

On the day scheduled for the interview bring a tape or digital recorder, and camera or camera phone as well as tablet of paper and several pens along. Invariable, like Murphy's Law and O'Toole's Corollary, one or two of the pens will run out of ink during the interview to your consternation and exasperation.

Before you start the interview officially, and while the recorder is on, ask your subject for permission to record the interview. This way you will have permission recorded along with the interview proper. Jot down main ideas that surface from responses to each question. Since you have the comfort of knowing you can review the recorded content at any time later, this allows you to maintain eye contact with your subject as he/she speaks. Your attention to your subject and interest in what he/she is saying is vital to maintaining energy during the interview and keeping your subject engaged in talking about his/her accomplishments to you, the interested observer.

Close the interview thanking your subject for his/her time and candidness. Ask permission to call again if you need further clarification on any part of what was discussed. Then leave at the appointed time.

Allow a few days to one week for the interview to gestate in your mind before attempting to write up the interview. When you do block out time for writing always allow blocks of at least four hours to be available undisturbed. Then...WRITE. Let the words spill out on paper without any censorship. Explore main points-limit to two or three main points-the remainder will be considered 'fill'. Do not enclose lists or make the interview sound like a manager's evaluation. Write the article in a magazine-type conversational style. Readers like to read articles that entertain as well as teach. Too much teaching starts to sound pompous to the reader and that is where you will lose them.

Over the next week or two, hopefully you will get a response from the Editor-in-Chief of the journal you hope to publish in. If it is a 'no' do not get discouraged- just write to another Editor-in-Chief of a different journal with your interview idea and keep on writing the article. Since you will be working on the article you will probably get one or two to responses from two separate editors because by then you will have completed the article and can send it along with a cover letter.

IMPORTANCE OF COVER LETTER

Remember this important fact-WHEN YOU SEND YOUR ARTICLE ACKNOWLEDGE THAT THE EDITOR DID NOT KNOW IT WAS COMING. The editor has no obligation to take his precious time in reading your article. BUT... if your cover letter has a compelling argument why the editor should read your article, and your writing style is at its best…you will be more likely to have your article read and even accepted. So, the morale of this section is- your best writing should take place in your cover letter in order to draw the editor's interest in reading more of what you have written.

INTERVIEW EXAMPLES

My first experience with interviewing a nurse-leader did not go well, but it was a good learning experience. My chosen nurse leader was a handicapped wheelchair-bound dean of a Midwestern School of Nursing. She had a Master's in Social Work (not nursing) and I felt that a non-nursing degree, plus her physical barriers made her an interesting candidate for an article on her leadership abilities in such an important and influential position. When I submitted the article to her for approval before sending it she was so critical of it that I lost interest in espousing all her great leadership qualities and just dropped the project at that point.

My second attempt went much better. I admired a nurse that I worked with in the Neonatal Intensive Care Unit (NICU) at a large Midwestern pediatric hospital. She had taken it upon herself to start a Parent's Support Group to help parents of babies in the NICU work through problems that they encountered. She came in on her own time two evenings a month to hold these meetings. In preparation, she would type up meeting time, date and invitation to attend, and post those invitations on the bed of every infant in the NICU. On the day of the meeting she would bake brownies or her special chocolate chip cookies to bring refreshment for the meeting attendees. This became especially important because many of the attendees were single parents who worked to maintain health [7]insurance and never seemed to have time or money to eat. They all enjoyed her baked goods. Also, upon finding out that their financial condition was so precarious and they did not get adequate meals, the nurse I interviewed convinced Hospital Administration to give breast-feeding mothers food coupons for two meals a day that could be used directly in the Hospital cafeteria. She maintained the argument that the meals would actually save the hospital money since the hospital did not have to provide formula for babies who were breast-fed. The reference for this article is as follows: [7, 8]

The third interview article practically wrote itself just by listening to my subject describe her life. Working within an extended care facility I became aware of the unusual background of the Director of Nurses. She had been a nurse missionary in China for 20 years before returning to the United States to resume practice here. I was intrigued wondering how she could balance her family and children's needs with her missionary nursing in a country whose language she did not know. This was probably the most fascinating of the interviews. I sat mesmerized and recorded as she spoke for two hours. That interview practically wrote itself from her words. [9] I only listened to the recording later while writing to check a fact or two.

Sredl, D. (2009). Janis Dickerman: A dream postponed, a destiny fulfilled. *Reflections on Nursing Leadership, 34*(4). (Electronic version).

My last two interviews were initiated for different reasons. One ultimately evolved into a published article. I asked to interview one of my colleagues in education for the purpose of nominating her for "Faculty of the Year Award" at our university. After extolling her numerous virtues, quite confident that her accomplishments, showcased in my writing, would earn her the reward she so richly deserved, I was astounded when the award was given to another faculty member who was facing a serious health concern. Unwilling to let perfectly good writing go to waste, I then started adapting my nomination letter into an article on leadership. With her patience and a very helpful and guiding Editor-in-Chief we saw that article in print by the end of the year. Instead of receiving recognition among 50 or so faculty at the university where we worked her talents and abilities were recognized by nurse scholars internationally. [9]

The outcome of my latest interview endeavor has just been resolved. I decided to nominate another of my education colleagues for a prestigious award given by the university. This was the Emerson Excellence in Teaching Award sponsored by Emerson Electric. This award had a lot of strings attached. First I had to tell my intended nominee of my plans to do this as it would require quite a bit of input directly from her. The nominee had to be a full time tenured professor with at least four years of teaching experience at this university. OK, given that, I needed to seek out letters of recommendation from six people: two from students; one from a colleague who had observed the nominee's classroom teaching, and three from respected community leaders who knew of the nominee's abilities. I found I needed to develop a checklist of my own to keep track of my sending out 'request for letters'; prompt to please write letter; and receipt of letter. Some of the prompts took 4-5 tries but I knew everybody I asked was in very busy and influential positions.

From the nominee I needed a CV, her teaching philosophy, and a summary of her evaluations from the last five years. My part involved securing all these documents in order to digest the content and sift out what I would use for the nomination letter, and to find examples of leadership activity as well as concrete EVIDENCE of the positive outcomes of her innovative teaching style.

This week the winner was announced…yes, my nominee won!

Photograph

As a would-be author, it is worth your time to contact a quality professional photographer, pick a sedate suit or other business casual attire and arrange (on a good hair day) a studio appointment for your professional photo. It may also be a good idea to pay the extra fee giving you copyright rights to *own* the photo so you can use it any time you want. Most publications will request a photo from you, the author, and you do not want to send them the one Grandma took of you in her backyard! A professional photograph is worth its weight in gold.

REFERENCES

[1]   Sredl, D., Response to 'The idea of nursing science' by S.D. Edwards (1999). *Journal of Advanced Nursing,* 2001. 35(3): p. 386-387.
[2]   Ellis, P., *The Essential Guide to Effect Sizes.* 2010, Cambridge, UK: Cambridge University Press.
[3]   Sredl, D., Sars: Here today and gone tomorrow? *Nursing Made Incredibly Easy* 2003. 1(2): p. 28-36.
[4]   Sredl, D., *More pressure sore treatment and why they're used.* RN, 1986. 1: p. 39.
[5]   Sredl, D., *Helping from my hospital bed.* RN, 2004. 67(3): p. 39-40.
[6]   Sredl, D., Danny. *Point of View,* 1994. 31(3): p. 2-3.
[7]   Sredl, D., *I saw a need.* Reflections on Nursing Leadership, 2003. Third Quarter: p. 30-32.
[8]   Sredl, D., Education of an educator. Reflections on Nursing Leadership-publication of STTI, 2014. 40(1).
[9]   Sredl, D., Janis Dickerman: A dream postponed, a destiny fulfilled. *Reflections on Nursing Leadership,* 2009. 34(4).

Chapter 4

PROFESSIONAL MANUSCRIPTS

It has been noted previously that the first step in any writing project is to actually sit down and WRITE! This may sound like an over-simplification but we all know people who say, "I could write a book…IF I had the time" in professing intimate knowledge of some topic, but the sad thing is- they rarely do. YOU can be different. Just block out some time (2-3 hours is a good rule of thumb), then start writing and don't censor yourself. I understand when you object, "Hey I am a busy person. I really don't have the time". Remember this-you always find the time for projects that you consider important. So, for you busy would-be writers who don't have the time but DO have a good idea that would make a block-buster article, I propose two methods to go about it. One is a semi-stall technique to gain more time called the query method. Here's how it works.

A. MANUSCRIPT VERSUS QUERY METHOD

There are two ways to go about gaining the Editor's interest in your writing. One, of course, is to submit an entire manuscript with a snazzy cover letter. If you have the time to research and develop your topic into a manuscript worthy of being called an article, then by all means do so. This is called 'the manuscript method'.

You can consult the internet for magazines/journals that provide a focus within the domain of your topic. Another way of finding the appropriate audience for your topic is to consult the 2014 (or current year's) Writer's Market. [1] This important reference text covers the contact information, main focus, and helpful tips to potential authors for their book or journal enterprise. It can be purchased for a reasonable sum in any bookstore or can be explored in the reference section of your local library. The Writer's Market contains a long list of US, Canadian and International book publishers, literary agents, consumer magazines trade journals, and even available contests and awards. Journal information includes payment per word/article; percent of issue that is freelance written; length of time for a decision; and tips for the writer new to that journal.

Photos often enhance article content and may even increase payment should your article be accepted. What no book will tell you…but I will tell you here …is that the only part of your writing that will actually be read at this stage is your cover letter. It has to be a SNAZZY cover letter leaving the editor wanting to read more. That editor wanting to read more will then move on to reading your article OR delegating the reading of your article to an assistant editor to get another point of view concerning your writing ability.

If the outcome of the editorial process is favorable and you receive an OK that your article will be published you are home-free. All you have to do is wait until you see your article published and then cash your check. But things do not usually turn out so well so fast in the publishing industry. Since technical/professional articles are so fact-filled, the editors who are already thinking favorably toward your article will then seek out two or three 'experts' in your field and ask them to review your article for accuracy, timeliness and overall potential reader interest. If the reviewers feel that the article is not appropriate for whatever reason, you will receive a letter from the editor that the article is being rejected. A rejection letter may not have anything to do with your writing or article development. The problem may be as simple as the fact that the journal covered a topic similar to yours within the past half-year. With a full rejection you are free to make changes you think appropriate and submit it to another journal. This is your lucky day!

IF, however, you receive a letter from the editor that says he/she likes the article but the reviewers found a few things that need to be changed- HALLELUYA! This, also, is your lucky day! Examine the reviewer's opinions carefully and revise the manuscript accordingly. It will undoubtedly be better as a result of the extra eyes on it. Ironically, however, this is when most writers fold up and fail. They become depressed and throw the manuscript in the circular file never to be sent out again. What they SHOULD realize is that their manuscript has already made it past the SNAZZY COVER LETTER test, past the interested editor, and on to the reviewers for comment. IF the editor did not think your article had potential (perhaps even, enormous potential) he/she would not already have invested so much time in it. So, as I said, make the changes that the reviewers recommended and submit the revised manuscript back by the recommended due date.

Sending Electronically

When you prepare to send your article electronically, whether it is first-time-out or a revision, it needs to be separated into parts so you will not go crazy trying to comply with directions at the time of submission. First, compose your SNAZZY COVER LETTER and save it as the topic and cover letter. For example, if I were writing about deer, I would save as 'Deer cover letter'. Then, in a similar manner prepare your title page by removing your name and contact information from it; copy and put it into a separate Word document, saving it as 'Deer title page'. You can easily see now how you need to separate into separate Word documents the Main article, references, tables (if any), and figures (if any).

When you register at the journal's website you will have to fill out a number of pages asking for contact information, position, work affiliation, etc. Then the page appears that asks you to browse your computer and upload in turn, your cover letter, title page (with identifying contact information removed), main manuscript, tables & figures (if any), and references. If you make a mistake, don't stress because you will also be able to re-order the documents you sent so that they will be in the proper order. The journal's processing center will convert your manuscript into one pdf document for your review. You may still make changes at this point. When you have reviewed your pdf and are satisfied with it, press the submit button. IT IS SENT!

Query Method

The second way to get published is to use the query method. There may be times when you have a great idea for an article but not enough time to develop it. You can still capture the Editor's attention and 'hold' a place for yourself by using the query method. This method involves composing a SNAZZY COVER LETTER (there's that phrase again), that briefly outlines your idea and points out YOUR CREDENTIALS that makes it most appropriate for YOU to write it and not one of their other staff writers. For example, maybe you have spliced together three types of roses to create a new hybrid. You took pictures of your new rose (always good to mention pictures as evidence when you have them) and, would be willing to include them with the manuscript when it is ready. You will either get a 'no' or a 'yes, go ahead-can you send by ___(date)_____?' Keep your time commitment and you just may have sold an article. All articles are on speculation with no firm commitment until you get the editor's message that the article has been ACCEPTED.

Royalties/Fees/Kill Fee

Book royalties, of course, are what every author lives for/hopes for…but they don't necessarily come easy. The royalty agreement is spelled out up front in the initial book contract that the author signs. It is usually a certain percentage of the book price for each copy sold…BUT…there is a caveat. Sometimes the royalty plan starts after a certain amount of books are sold royalty-free in order for the publisher to recoup some of their administrative, copy-editing, and printing costs. For example, the agreement may read, 8% royalty on each book sold after the first 200 books are sold. The publisher may issue annual, quarterly or semi-annual statements of books sold and royalty earned.

Articles in professional journals are a different story. Most professional journals do not pay for articles. It is considered prestige to be published in the top, well-respected journals. Bylines of author names and institutions represented are always included with the article. With hard copy journals this is usually sufficient and no money passes hands one way or the other.

Open Access

Open access publications are relatively new on the publishing scene. These are essentially professional e-zines that do not require subscriptions. The 'open access' means that anyone can look up the article via Pubmed or one of the other databases and, without having an affiliation or subscription to that journal can download the article for free. While this article access is free to the person who wants the article, it is not free to the author, or institution the author represents. Since the journal is online with no printed matter the journal cannot take in money to pay expenses from advertisers such as a printed journal can. So…it charges the author whose article is accepted a fee. That fee can range from $200 to $1100 USD. One might be tempted to think that any author can get published by paying the fee but that is not true. The open access journals go through the same peer-review process that print journals require. This means that not only editorial approval is needed, but also of the two or three experts that the editor sends your article out to review. Only then, if approval is unanimous, does the journal deem your article good enough to be 'accepted' and ask for the open access fee. It is a good idea to build an 'open-access publication fee' into the grant budget. Then you will have set the stage for publication AND paying the open access fee if your article gets accepted even a year or two after the grant is approved.

Kill Fee

This doesn't happen too often but it may happen to you so let's discuss it here. Sometimes an editor makes a commitment to accept an article...then...probably because they are so busy...forgets about it. The journal has made the commitment to accept the article, so legally the journal must keep it's concomitant commitment to pay you, the author, but it doesn't have to publish your article. This is known as a publisher paying a'kill fee'. Kill fees can also work in reverse too.

Once I received an authorization to publish my article 'New Therapies for Decubitus Ulcer Management'. I forgot about it until one day while sorting a stack of papers on my credenza I came across the acceptance letter. Two years had passed and now many of the therapies I wrote about as 'new' were in actuality already being used and not considered new at all. My professional reputation was on the line, I felt. So, I wrote to the Editor and sent a copy of the acceptance letter asking them not to use the article since the therapies were no longer new. Soon a letter of apology arrived asking if I would consider a $200 kill fee for their mistake. I said I would--send the check! You can imagine my amazement when a few months later that journal came out with an issue that looked like a Playboy centerfold! It was indeed a centerfold in 4-color glossy paper of a stage 4 decubitus ulcer! Around the picture were text boxes from seven different authors. Since my name was among them, I read on. The text box with my material contained two paragraphs from my original article. I assumed that the other six authors had also written about decubitus ulcers. Since I had accepted the kill fee, technically the manuscript was theirs to do with as they wished. They wished up a compelling centerfold with vignettes from seven authors. Ingenious!

B. DISSERTATION

Although every graduate student aspiring to the doctorate has a dissertation committee and chair to guide his/her work through the dissertation writing process, I do have one tip that may not be covered and may prove very helpful to the student.

That Tip Is This: Choose a Topic That Can Be Researched As Quickly and Cheaply As Possible

Plan to pay for any expense involved yourself rather than writing a grant application and waiting for the IRB committee to approve/disapprove it at their quarterly meeting. This lengthy process never guarantees that a grant will be funded and you can easily lose 1-2 YEARS in the waiting process. Some estimates have determined that the median cost to research and write a dissertation is $1500. Your costs, however, may be substantially below this if you do not have to pay an honorarium for use of an established research instrument; use Survey Monkey™ or some other internet response service instead of mailing questionaires via US Postal Service.

Ironically most students do not heed this advice, and as a result many never complete the dissertation writing process at all forever listing ABD (all but dissertation) instead of Ph.D. after their name. I theorize that one of the reasons for this is because the student is so intent on researching a topic so novel, so compelling, that he/she is willing to sacrifice speed –to-graduation for novelty. **Don't do this!** Graduate and get that degree first; *then* you can go on at the higher income level to research any esoteric and/or hard- to- find- evidence- on- topics that you wish to study. By then you will have a faculty position at a prestigious university and all the faculty help to assist you in studying your topic of special interest.

Let me give you an example of what I mean. I am also a certified hypnotherapist. I was interested in Eye Movement Dissociation Response (EMDR) and it's relationship to hypnosis. I wanted to research the similarities and differences between the two techniques. I was in private hypnosis practice with my own office and thought I could draw participants from my clientele for the study with their informed consent. The chair of my committee approved this and also stated that multi-site studies were favored for grants.

So, now I was thinking I would have to get hypnosis-certified in one or two more states and try to get patients in those states. Then I remembered that in order to obtain study participants I would have to get Institutional Review Board approval from each of the hospital/medical centers in those two states. My recent experience with gaining IRB approval for a study in my own state took 9 months. Then, I started worrying about air fare and accommodation expenses. I would have to write a grant to secure the funds to undertake this study. Worse still, I knew from my own hypnosis practice experience that many times patients (and, I theorized that possibly study participants might also) cancel their appointments with little notice. I envisioned being in a strange city to see one study participant only to find the participant had a change of heart and cancelled the study appointment. I had nightmares over the financial, physical and emotional toll this research might bring upon me and my family. I began to doubt that I would ever finish the dissertation and obtain my Ph.D. I wondered why my dissertation chair and committee let me pursue this absurd idea.

Then a wonderful thing happened. By chance (or, maybe not by chance-sometimes miracles are coincidences in which God chooses to remain anonymous) I interviewed for a job with one person who had also been a student in one of the Ph.D. classes that I was also in. She told me that she had done her research and wrote her dissertation in one year! I asked how she did that, thinking of all the convoluted twists and turns that my own research presented. She told me she focused on symptoms of asthma; mailed a questionnaire to fifty asthma patients who met inclusion criteria in the doctor's office where she worked; did simple central tendency statistics and, got her degree. Amazing! And, wonderful advice. I didn't get that job- after all I didn't have my Ph.D. yet. But I did change my focus, designed a new and much simpler study, and went on to get my Ph.D. Yes, I am doing more complicated research now but with plenty of highly qualified faculty colleagues to assist.

Dissertation Template

The usual arrangement of chapters in a dissertation is a **template** as follows: ***Chapter One-topic and study design; Chapter Two- Literature Review; Chapter Three-Methodology; Chapter Four- Statistical Analysis; Chapter Five- Discussion***. You will find many fine books exploring dissertation completion; American Psychological Association (APA), and American Medical Association (AMA) style formats; etc. Read one or more of them to help organize your thoughts but remember my tip before you begin the process.

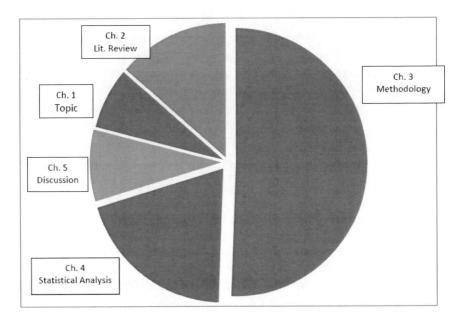

Figure/Template 4-1. Dissertation.

Chapter One-topic and study design; Chapter Two- Literature Review; Chapter Three-Methodology; Chapter Four- Statistical Analysis; Chapter Five- Discussion.

C. GRANT WRITING

Research costs money. So, it behoves us to discuss grant writing before we discuss clinical research. To begin, writing an excellent grant (here we mean the word 'excellent' to be synonymous with the word 'funded') also means that the entire methodology of the proposed study must previously be thought out because explaining the methodology along with identifying a need for the result of this study is necessary. Also necessary is a detailed budget for the requested amount of funds.

It is beyond the expertise of this author to discuss National Institutes of Health research grants, but I can discuss non-national, non- government grants that are within reach. There are certain similarities that comprise the **template** of every grant funding agency.

Searching for Funding

Foundations are often good sources of funds *IF their preferred funding correlates well with your proposed topic.* You should look up the composition of the funding agency because some foundations only employ 1 person; some employ none at all and just award the required amount of annual funding to one or more educational endeavors of their choice. Do not waste your time (and theirs) by trying to influence their decision-making to include your topic for funding within their established funding plan. Public libraries in some large cities may have a Foundation section which includes the names and funding focus of various foundations.

Non-profit hospitals usually have a philanthropic arm that includes foundation funds for special projects. So, if you plan to submit a grant application to one of these healthcare institutions, your research methodology rationale should also include how your proposed research will benefit the hospital. Remember to include 'open access publication fee' in your grant budget.

IRB

Grant applications are also looked upon more favorably if the hospital's *Institutional Review Board (IRB)* has approved your request for the research. Here again your methodology for the study must already be firmly established in order to gain IRB approval. These boards usually meet quarterly, so if the IRB application is not approved, it may be sent back to you with comments from the reviewers so that you can amend and resubmit it before the deadline for the next meeting.

When the IRB has approved your study, they will stamp an approval number on your IRB application face sheet which is the number you should use on your grant application.

The first page or two of the grant application should read like a literature review and incorporate main points of interest why this research NEEDS to be done. Always proceed from the general to the very specific, like pouring liquid through a funnel-large opening to small. After the generalities of why you want to do this study you must then make a solid case as to why you are applying to *this* funding source for operating funds. Maybe you have identified a need for motorized wheelchairs for patients who are veterans with amputated lower limbs and this hospital has a large PT/OT department and clientele of disabled veterans. This research focus would probably be a good match for the facility's need. The methodology, or how specifically you plan to proceed with the study needs to be explained next. Contact information for you, as the primary investigator, and any others assistants who will have access to the data need to be listed next. A copy of the Informed Consent (and Parent Assent Agreement if children are required participants) needs to be included as well as an explanation of how the potential participant was allowed to question the researcher. Finally, the detailed budget must be developed that identifies where every dollar that you are asking for is planned to be spent. In-kind services, office space & equipment must also be included as a percentage of the total amount.

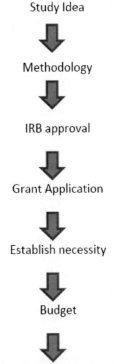

Study Idea

Methodology

IRB approval

Grant Application

Establish necessity

Budget

Expected Outcomes (reasons why funding agency should want to fund this study)

Figure/Template 4-2. Grant Template.

Clinical Research Article

Clinical research articles yield the latest evidence on any given topic. This is why researchers try to get the results of their clinical trials published as quickly as possible after study completion. Unlike books that may take up to five years to get published, articles can go through the reviewer process in three to six months and be published within one year of study completion. This ascertains that the very latest research information is available at the earliest opportunity. Clinical trial study findings are considered the 'gold standard' of evidence by those espousing evidence-based medical practice. However, having said that, I must also say that no one study 'proves' anything. Findings discussions can only yield results from a specified pool of participants and may not be generalized to the population at large. Similarly it is first and foremost among the six levels of evidence that nurses examine.

EBP Levels of Evidence

The evIdence-based process typically contains data from several sources including: empirical research, patient history, assessment and goals, nursing expertise at all levels (DNP, Ph.D., APN, consultants, expert panels, etc), available resources and qualitative studies.

The ABSTRACT is of utmost importance when beginning to consolidate data from a research study. Interested readers want a thumbnail sketch of what the article is initially about without having to read the entire article. They want to know more about the study, the hypotheses/research questions, and findings and relevance to their profession. From this information they can tell if the article meets or matches their inclusion criteria for their own project, be that a literature review or integrative literature review. Non research articles or opinion papers can host an abstract of a mere 40 words, but a research study demands a formal format of 300 words with the following template of inclusions.

Clinical Relevance

The body of the article includes additional qualifiers such as statistical relevance, strengths and weaknesses, and possibly ethical considerations.

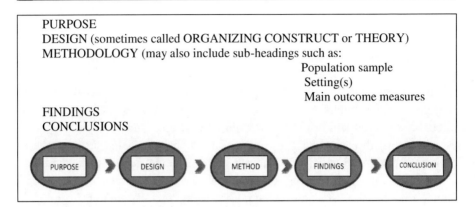

Figure/Template 4-3. Clinical Research Template.

Impact Factor

One important consideration as you try to decide which professional journal that you want to see your article published in is that journal's IMPACT FACTOR. The impact factor reflects the journal's importance and potential readership. The closer it is to '2', the higher the impact factor. Realistically, if the journal's impact factor is 1.647 (for example) it is a highly respected and sought after journal.

D. CONCEPT ANALYSIS

Concept Analysis-How to Do It

Concepts are the building blocks or, BRICKS of theory development. The hypotheses, relationships & relational statements are the MORTAR of theory development that glues it all together. The theory itself is the BLUEPRINT of the entire project (Sredl, 2006). Their primary function: To examine the basic elements of a concept in order to distinguish that concept from others that are similar **but not the same.**

*Results of concept analysis***: provides the scientist with an excellent beginning for a new tool or an excellent way to evaluate an old one.** Since concepts may have completely different meanings in different theoretical venues, it is incumbent upon nursing scholars to provide concept analysis for the nursing literature.

Adapted from, Walker, O., & Avant, K. (2005). *Strategies for Theory Construction in Nursing.* (4ᵗʰ Ed.).

Writing a concept analysis may be one of the simplest and most rewarding types of writing for three reasons. First, there is an established template that guides the format of the analysis; second, the analysis combines fiction and non-fiction, and; third it furthers the case of nursing research by defining a term or phrase that can be used in experimental as well as quasi-experimental studies. Let's begin by asking a series of questions...

What is a concept? Concepts are mental constructions of our attempts to provide order to our environmental stimuli.

What do concepts contain? Concepts contain categories of information that contain defining characteristics/attributes that make up the concept.

What is the purpose of a concept analysis: To "get inside" a concept & see how it works; to understand how the concept contains *within itself* the attributes or characteristics that make it unique from other concepts; to encourage communication & promote understanding among our colleagues about the particular phenomena discussed. The process of concept analysis, then, is a formal, linguistic exercise to discover those defining attributes by careful description of a word and how it is 'like' and 'not like' other closely related words or terms.

There are three types of concept analyses: normal, hybrid, and evolutionary. We will discuss all three but for the purposes of this text we will concentrate on the normal concept analysis since it is the one most commonly used.

Template for Normal Concept Analysis

The template involves writing an introduction developing a case for why you feel a concept analysis should be done. Once you have established the necessity you can go on to identify the CRITICAL ATTRIBUTES of the word or phrase. Critical attributes, as the name suggests are those qualities that comprise the very meaning of the word/phrase and MUST BE associated with the word/phrase in every context that it is used. I have found it most helpful to use a table with five columns using the following headings: ANTECEDENT, CRITICAL ATTRIBUTES, CONSEQUENCES (sometimes called DETERMINANTS), EMPIRICAL REFERENTS, AND INSTRUMENT(s). It should look like this:

Concept Analysis Worksheet

Antecedent	Critical Attribute	Consequence	Empirical referent	Instrument

Figure/Template 4-4. Concept Analysis Worksheet.

You can copy this template and use it for all your brainstorming sessions. The following is an abbreviated example that will be used and filled-in when describing the steps to take in developing the analysis. We begin by identifying the concept of "LOVE".

Concept: Love

Antecedent	Critical attribute	Consequences	Empirical referent	Instrument

Figure/Template 4-5. Concept of LOVE.

Begin by brainstorming the second column. Without censoring yourself, try to think of as many creative ways to describe the word/phrase you are analyzing. **Begin by working on the second column first**. Find all the 'critical attributes' that absolutely MUST be considered as integral parts of the concept. If you can trim down to one or two words or a short phrase, it can be listed in the second column. I have found it useful to identify All the critical attributes before working on any of the other columns.

The editing of this process will come later when you find you cannot fill the other columns with appropriate identifiers. The most important thing to consider at this point is finding enough qualifiers that absolutely *have to be present* within the word you are analyzing. Let's assume we are analyzing the concept of 'LOVE'. One possible critical attribute of love is 'emotional attachment'.

Antecedent	Critical attribute	Consequences	Empirical referent	Instrument
	Emotional Attachment			

Figure/Template 4-6. First step- Critical Attribute.

Next, we go back to the first column. Looking at the critical attribute of 'emotional attachment' in the second column we think about what might have come first. What might have preceded (ante- meaning before) emotional attachment' to qualify as LOVE? Possibly the phrase "satisfying personal relationship" might be expected to come before the 'emotional attachment'? When all the critical attributes have been identified you may move toward completing the first column, the Antecedent. This first column looks at the critical attribute and identifies what came *first* toward developing that critical attribute. For example, if the critical attribute were 'LOVE", the antecedent may be 'Heartfelt emotion'.

Antecedent	Critical attribute	Consequences	Empirical referent	Instrument
Satisfying Personal Relationship	Emotional attachment			

Figure/Template 4-7. Second step-Antecedent.

If so, then what comes as a result? We look to the third column asking, what is the consequence of a 'satisfying personal relationship' that has led to an 'emotional attachment'? Next we work on the third column, the 'Consequence'. If 'heartfelt emotion' led to 'LOVE', then a consequence of LOVE might be 'good feelings toward another person', or another consequence might be 'physical contact'.

Antecedent	Critical attribute	Consequences	Empirical referent	Instrument
Satisfying Personal Relationship	Emotional attachment	Physical contact		

Figure/Template 4-8. Third step-Consequences.

If we then accept a consequence of 'physical contact' we can assume any number of empirical referents, which are examples of the consequence. For example, the 'physical contact' might be manifested by a 'kiss' or a 'handshake', or even 'intercourse'. Any of those words could describe a "satisfying personal relationship that has led to an emotional attachment manifested by the physical contact of a kiss". The fourth column, or empirical referent' is the **physical manifestation** of the Critical Attribute. In our example of LOVE as a critical attribute we might see "kiss' as one of those manifestations.

You have now completed one row across the critical attribute table.

Antecedent	Critical attribute	Consequences	Empirical referent	Instrument
Satisfying Personal Relationship	Emotional attachment	Physical contact	Kiss	

Figure/Template 4-9. Fourth step Empirical Referent.

Finally, the fifth column is the research instrument that can be used to measure the critical attribute.

Here is an example of a completed concept analysis on Thermostability from the 5-concept analyses supporting the Aerohemodynamics Theory as first identified in 1983 in:

Sredl, D. (1983). *Airborne Patient Care Management: A Multidisciplinary Approach.* St. Louis, Medical Research Associates.
(Translated into Spanish and adopted by the Government of Chile as their official Air Evacuation Manual.)

Concept Analysis –Thermostability

Antecedent	Critical Attribute	Consequence	Empirical referent	Instrument
Heating/cooling Element	Temperature	Heat/cool	Thermometer	Thermometer
Space	Environment	Surroundings	Living space	area
No equilibrium	equilibrium	homeostasis	Calmness	No discernible change
Ambient equilibrium	Heat	Boiling	Steam	Thermometer
No tension	Stress	> tension	> anxiety	> HR, RR, & BP
Instability	Stability	Equilibrium	Homeostasis	No discernible change
Thermal Instability	Ambient	Equilibrium	Homeostasis	No discernible change
Ambient equilibrium	Boil	Steam	Steam	Thermometer
Cold	Freeze	Ice	Ice	Thermometer
Ambience	Thermal	Temperature Measurement	Thermometer	thermometer
Liquid	Steam	Condensation	Water molecules Visible in air	Thermometer
Solid mass	Vaporization	Spatial Molecular Escape	Water molecules Visible in air	Water molecules Visible in air
Cold water	Ice	Water Molecular Expansion	Ice	Visualization of Expanded Water
Cold water	Icecicles	Gravity-dir-Ected frozen Water	Tubular hanging Ice	Visualization of Expanded water

(Continued)

Antecedent	Critical Attribute	Consequence	Empirical referent	Instrument
Cold water	**Glacier**	**Water frozen** Into large block Of ice	**Massive ice**	**Visualization of** Expanded **Water**
High humidity	**Avalanche**	**Destructive snow** Path	**Snow flow**	**Visualization of** Large mass snow flow
High humidity	**Snow**	**Frozen water** Crystals	**Floating ice** Crystals	**Visualization of** ice
Glacial ice Intact	**Ice-berg**	**Ice floating in** Water	**Ice floes in** Water	**Visualization of** Expanded **Water**
No combustion	**Fire**	**Mass destroyed**	**Flame**	**Flames visible**
Neutral temp-erature	**Vaporization**	**Water droplets** Suspended in Air	**Water molecules** Visible in air	**Water molecules Visible in air**
Neutral Temperature	**Combustion**	**Fire**	**Fire**	**Flames visible**

Figure/Template 4-10. Completed Concept analysis graphic of Thermostability.
(Reprinted with permission of Elsevier).

Completion of the fifth column (if you can) is the icing on the cake. That column identifies a recognized research instrument that can be used to MEASURE some facet of the critical attribute, 'Emotional attachment'. A concept analysis does not have to have the fifth column completed in order to be a valuable addition to research vocabulary-it is optional.

How Concept Analysis Is Helpful in Theory

1) Concept analysis refines ambiguous words in a theory
2) It clarifies overused words so that everybody speaks/thinks of the same thing.
3) It results in an operational definition that increases the validity of the construct.

4) Results of concept analysis yield a basic understanding of the underlying attributes of the concept, which aids in theory development
5) Clarifies defining problems
6) Allows the theorist to construct hypotheses that accurately reflect the relationships between/among concepts.
7) Results of concept analysis are useful indicators to use when formulating research instruments or establishing questions for field interview guides prior to conducting research, or in evaluating the validity of existing instruments.

Important note- Language changes it's meanings from time to time. There is a dynamic quality of ideas that may change along with, or independent of changes in vocabulary. Ex: the word "cool" at one time was a representation of temperature. Over time it came into common usage as slang to indicate something (anything) that was considered "good".

What Is the Step- by- Step Procedure for a Concept Analysis

(These steps are adapted from Wilson"s 11 steps (1963) and re-adapted from Walker & Avant's 8 steps (2005).

1) Select a concept
2) Determine the aims or purpose of the analysis in the introduction.
3) Identify any & all primary uses of the concept that you can.
4) Determine the defining attributes-the important words that make up the *essence* of the concept

(Now comes the fictional part of the concept analysis!)

1. Construct a model case in which the concept and ALL of the identified Critical Attributes play a part. *(Be prepared to identify these Critical Attributes by underlining, italicizing, or emboldening them directly after the attribute appears in the model case in order to make it easier for the reader to see that the model case does indeed encompass ALL the Critical Attributes.)*

2. Identify borderline, related, contrary, invented, and illegitimate cases;
    Think of the following scenarios that the concept may play a different
    part in:

    a. Borderline case- it might be used in and contains MOST of
        the defining attributes, but not all of them;
    b. A related case- a case that demonstrates ideas similar to the
        main concept but actually differs when closely examined;
    c. A contrary case- a clear example of a situation that does not
        demonstrate the concept. It does not necessarily have to
        demonstrate qualities opposite of the identified attributes of
        the concept under discussion, but rather show that the
        concept with its previously described attributes does not exist
        in this particular situation;An invented case-is one that
        contains ideas outside our actual experience. Take the
        concept out of its ordinary environment & place it in another
        context entirely. Not all concept analyses include this step-
        but it is fun to let your creativity loose!
    d. An illegitimate case is one that uses the concept out of
        context. Most of the attributes that you defined will not apply
        in this scenario.

Once the cases have been put together, compare them to the defining
attributes to ensure that all defining attributes have been discovered.
"AN ANALYSIS IS NOT COMPLETE UNTIL THERE ARE NO
OVERLAPPING ATTRIBUTES AND NO CONTRADICTIONS BETWEEN
THE DEFINING ATTRIBUTES AND THE MODEL CASE" Walker &
Avant, 2005).

3. Identify antecedents and consequences.

    a. *Antecedents* (sometimes called *"determinants"* in the
        literature) are those events or incidents that must occur prior
        to the occurrence of the concept. Helpful in identifying
        underlying assumptions regarding the concept. Ex. In the
        concept of "pregnancy"- one antecedent might be "ovulation"
    b. *Consequences* are events or incidents that occur as a result of
        the occurrence of the concept. Helpful in identifying
        neglected ideas, variables or relationships that may yield
        NEW research directions. Ex. In the concept of "pregnancy"-
        one consequence might be "delivery"

4. Define empirical referents of the concept. Empirical referents are examples of actual phenomena that, by their very existence, demonstrate the occurrence of the concept itself. Ask the question, "If this concept exists, how can we measure it? Empirical referents are useful in theory development because they are linked to the theoretical base of the concept. Example – the concept of "affection" one empirical referent might be "kissing" (Sometimes the defining attribute and the empirical referent will be identical.)

Following the completion of the worksheet you may proceed to let your imagination run wild as you enter the fiction phase of concept analysis-Constructed Cases.

The following are constructed cases as suggested by Walker and Avant [2]. The first constructed case is the model case that contains *all* of the critical attributes identified comprising the concept under study. In the following example each critical attribute is identified by italics. They may also be identified by underlining or emboldening them.

Model Case

Dr. Harvey was a well- respected physician employed in the radiation therapeutics department of a large Midwestern hospital. She had a *depth* of experience with many different types of *radiation dosing* including *X-rays, Gamma-rays, ultraviolet, ultrasound, microwave* emissions and even *rad* exposure to such technical instruments as airline *sound communication, radio transponder* and *emergency locator transmission (ELT)*. Dr Harvey was called upon to testify as an expert witness during many court cases involving *frequency* of *exposure* to skin cancer caused by the sun's *rays*- even through *clouds* and *sun-block* lotion.

Contrary Case

The elderly couple from the Midwest decided to vacation in the Bahamas. Because of the negative publicity about skin damage caused by the sun, the couple spent the duration of their vacation playing cards in their darkened hotel room.

Advantages and Limitations of Concept Analysis

There are both strengths and limitations, advantages and pitfalls, to a concept analysis. Among the advantages are a clarification of language, symbols, words and terms. By defining precisely what the word or phrase means, researchers can have a common starting understanding for variable terms that they can use in theoretical and operational definitions for theory construction and research. Concept analysis clarifies nursing terms that have become 'catchphrases' and/or have lost exact meaning while adding professionalism to nursing language development. Concept analysis encourages critical thinking and is helpful in research instrument identification and/or development.

Limitations of concept analysis include succumbing to the pitfall that concept analysis is too easy-or conversely that you are in over your head. Concept analysis is a new way of thinking that may require some getting used to in the beginning leading to the compulsion to analyze everything. There is also the author's temptation to moralize when the concept under analysis has value implications.

How Are Concept Analyses Used in the Development or Affirmation of Nursing Theory?

Concepts Are the Building Blocks of Theory

Conceptual Models of Nursing Theory
Conceptual models, sometimes equated with Grand Theory, are statements of general, comprehensive and often abstract perspectives of the nursing paradigm. The observation propositions comprising a conceptual model are not themselves empirically measurable therefore they depend upon the variables analyzed in concept analyses to provide more clarity to the conceptual model. Because of this conceptual models are not directly applicable in a clinical situation, but their generality means they can be applied to everybody.

Middle Range Theory
Middle range nursing theory differs from the abstraction of grand theory primarily in that in cannot be applied to everybody, but rather an identified segment of society, such as children. Utilizing concepts analyzed by Walker &

Avant's technique, middle range theory has incorporated the tools of concrete language defined in measurable ways that can be directly applied in clinical situations. Hypotheses stating specific and observable relationships can better predict phenomena that might influence particular behaviors in specific research studies.

Concept Analysis Hybrid, Evolutionary and Wilsonian

Hybrid
Primary function: To identify various approaches to measure concepts of interest to nursing.

These approaches are based on knowledge from 3 bodies of literature:

1) Philosophy of science
2) Field research methods
3) Sociology of theory construction

The theoretical and empirical perspectives are combined to focus on the concept's definition and measurement & relies heavily on insights generated from clinical practice.

There are 4 phases of hybrid concept analysis:

1. *Theoretical phase with extensive review of literature.* This phase focuses on identifying the essential elements of the concept, developing an initial working definition and considering the concept's
2. Measurement potential.
3. *Fieldwork phase that generates clinically based empirical data describing the concept.* This phase works to uncover:
   - In what ways is the concept conveyed to patients by healthcare professionals?
   - How are interactions utilized by this concept described?
4. *Analytical phase which synthesizes theoretical and empirical findings to validate and finalize concepts definition and key indicators (critical attributes* (Brown, 1997). In this phase findings from both the theoretical and fieldwork phase are combined to ask…

Figure/Template 4-11A. Hybrid Concept Analysis.

- How significant and applicable is the concept to the groups that were studied?
- Have the key indicators (critical attributes) changed over the course of the study?
- Has the definition changed?
- Is the concept measurable?

The write-up may include a table of **CONCEPTUAL INDICATORS, BEHAVIORAL INDICATORS, AND OPERATIONAL INDICATORS**

Conceptual indicators	Behavioral indicators	Operational indicators

Figure/Template 4-11B.

Evolutionary Concept Analysis

Primary function: To identify that a concept is constantly changing or "evolving" Rodgers (1989; 2000 a, b) says that "the idea behind the concept is of importance, not necessarily the term itself." Rodgers also cited the evolutionary concept analysis process as "a dynamic cycle with three cyclical influences":

1) Significance- identification of concept characteristics (critical attributes) that are hallmarks of the concept.
2) Use – referents, antecedents and consequences of the concept.
3) Application- implications for nursing practice

Steps in Evolutionary Concept Analysis

1) Identify concept of interest
2) Identify surrogate terms and relevant uses
3) Identify and select appropriate sample (minimum of 20%) of identified literature from relevant discipline using a systematic approach and broad time frame.
4) Identify attributes of concept

5) Identify antecedents, consequences and referents of concept if possible.
6) Identify related concepts
7) Identify a model (or "real") case of the concept

Figure/Template 4-12. Evolutionary Concept Analysis.

This method helps to clarify and develop concepts rather than describe their essence!

Review of Steps in Wilsonian Concept Analysis (Wilson, 1963) Walker and Avant, 2005

1) Select a concept
2) Determine the aims or purpose of analysis
3) Identify all uses of the concept that you can discover
4) Determine the defining attributes
5) Identify a model case
6) Identify contrary, borderline, related, invented, and illegitimate cases
7) Identify antecedents and consequences
8) Define empirical referents.

Figure/Template 4-13. Wilsonian Concept Analysis (normal).

Working through steps is an iterative process, not necessarily sequential. See p 63-84 Walker & Avant, 2005

Meta-Analysis

The crème de la crème of research writing is to be found within the realm of meta-analysis researchers. We said earlier that one research study ***does not prove anything!***

What about two or three with similar conclusions, you may be asking--- NOPE- still does not prove anything. BUT...what about hundreds of studies with findings of similar conclusions-does that make a difference? Hum-m-m...now we may be getting somewhere.

A meta-analysis is an integrative review of it's own type of research with an hypothesis, inclusion/exclusion criteria, and identified variables that is statistically analyzed for EFFECT SIZE. As Paul Ellis says in his text on how to calculate effect sizes, many research studies do not pass the "so what" test.

They may interpret the statistical significance of their results but rarely interpret their results in ways that are significant to non-statisticians.

After a thorough literature review is completed you will be ready to code the variables so that the data-points can be statistically analyzed by a parametric test that a power-analysis will indicate is the most powerful for the study. Effect sizes are, in effect, the meaning about research results. It still does not prove anything but rather, gives you, the reader, a scholarly estimation of how large an effect this combination of variables can have in real life.

When you master the writing of a meta-analysis you have mastered one of the most difficult forms of writing! Kudos to you, dear Writer!

Personal Helps

Resume Writing

Developing your resume sounds like a fairly simple task at first-after all who knows you better than YOU? But, putting the best information together in a one page document that the friendly folks in Human Resources wish to hire takes a little time to get it right. This like all the other forms of writing we have previously explored lends itself well to a template. The preferred format looks like this:

Contact information at the top in bold Objective Education: Highest degree earned first (ABSOLUTELY NO HIGH SCHOOL if you have a college degree or work toward it) Present Position Previous Positions Honors & Awards/ Special skills References available upon request

Figure/Template 4-14- Resume

Contact Information

Let's go over each category and expand upon it a little. The contact information is the Human Resource professional's first look at YOUR professionalism. Pay special attention to your email address and if it seems inappropriate (like perhaps, hot Moma @ gmail.com) get another one that will be used exclusively for resume submission and responses. Likewise be careful of how you record your phone voice mail greeting. Although it is cute to have your puppy bark "Hello" or have one of your children say something, it is a big turn-off when a Human Resource professional hears it. Change to a professional greeting in a professional tone and demeanor.

Objective

Here is where you identify your dream job. If you are an RN and want to secure a job at _____Hospital as an RN-say so! The Human Resources professionals spend less than one minute on average reading, sorting & making call-back decisions on resumes. ONE MINUTE!!! You want to use that minute to your advantage. Tell them up front what position you are seeking.

Education

Place your highest degree first. You may also put your grade point average if you choose to do so if it is admirable (perhaps over 3.0 on a 4.0 scale). You may also indicate a graduation date if in the near future and the degree that graduation will earn for you. Unless you are just starting out and have only a high school education, it is advisable to not put your high school down.

Present Position

Identify your present position and where you are employed. If you have done anything outstanding you may also list it here, but do not be too effusive.

Previous employment

Past positions may be listed if you think you will receive a good reference from the previous employer. If not do not include it but be aware that large gaps in work history will probably be expected to be explained in the interview. Include positions such as 'bartender' or 'waitress' which can be points to discuss transferrable skills.

Honors and Awards/ Special skills

Any type of special skills can be included here. If you made Dean's list. If you speak a language other than English list it here in bold.

References

Conclude the resume by the simple sentence- "References available upon request". Have a separate sheet prepared with the contact information of three references that you have previously asked permission to include. You respect your references too much to just have anybody look at their contact information, so, when you get the interview opportunity-that's when you release the separate sheet with all their contact information.

Curriculum Vitae

The phrase, 'Curriculum Viitae' (CV), derives from the Latin meaning curriculum of life. Like it sounds the CV is supposed to cover all professional endeavors in the life of the individual. It, rather than the resume, is mainly utilized for academic appointments. Just as the resume was considered optimal if condensed to 1 page, the CV is considered the more expansive the better. Here is a template that may be used to begin to develop a CV but modifications are welcome.

CV Template

Contact information

Education

Present position

Previous positions (ALL)

Military status

Professional organizations and offices held

Publications-(these may be separated into specific categories such as refereed publications; data-based publications; abstracts; books; book chapters; podium presentations)

Service and percentage of time:

Community

University

Courses taught including independent study

Acted as Committee Chair for the following students (date):

Acted as Committee member for the following students (date):

Honors and Awards

Figure/Template 4-15 CV.

Book

Perhaps the most important writing/publishing achievement most authors and would-be authors long for is the publication of their own book. This is often evidenced by comments such as "I could write a book about...if I had the time." This kind of thinking is synonymous with saying, "I could be a millionaire...if I had the money". So could we all! Achievements do not come without a concomitant amount of work.

If you have a special interest in a particular topic, start researching all angles of it. Talk to people about it in order to get new (and possibly hidden [from you] perspectives about it). Jot down notes as inspiration hits. I recommend keeping a note-pad and pen under your bed to instantly catch those inspiring thoughts as you wake no matter the time. You may think you will remember them later; but, you won't.

When you feel that you have enough material to make a case for a publishing company to accept your idea and offer you a contract for a book, use the template for proposing a "Book Idea" such as the one enclosed by this publishing company with permission.

If a contract is offered it will specify how long the publisher expects to wait before receiving your completed manuscript; the advance (if any); royalty percentage; and any other information relative to the publication. Some publishers expect to sell a certain number of books royalty- free before your royalty payment starts. This is understandable considering all the copy-editing work and paper, ink and printing expenses that the publisher incurs as a result of agreeing to publish your idea. Keep your time commitment! This means setting aside a certain amount of time each day to write. I print out a number of sheets-each with a part of a chapter and the expected date of completion for it. Then I tape each sheet to a wall in my house that is readily accessible-bedroom or kitchen. If I taped them to my office wall I would find too many excuses not to enter my office-but there is no getting away from entering and seeing them on either the kitchen or bedroom wall.

As I complete my self-imposed writing projects I rip that sheet down and can proceed to the next. Sometimes I write them out of order if I am particularly interested in one over the other as I know I can always reassemble them later. The last sheet of paper should say, "REVISE, REVISE, REVISE".

Then do it! And...you will soon be an author, my friend!

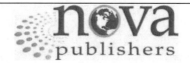

BOOK IDEA FORM

For Monographs or Edited Collections Proposals

Please Return to: n.columbus@novapublishers.com

Please Type in Subject Line of your Email: BIF for monograph or edited collection attached
Decision will be sent within 30 days of receipt
Average production cycle 28 weeks for hardcover books and 120 days for softcover
Books can be updated and revised at 6, 12 and 18 months after first publication date

Date: _____

Provisional title of the proposed publication:

_____

Type of publication proposed:
_____ **Monograph:** A monograph is a specialist original work of writing on a single subject or an aspect of a subject, usually by a single author (co-authors welcome).
_____ **Edited Collection:** A collection of scholarly or scientific chapters written by different authors collected together in one book by an editor(s). The chapters in an edited volume are original works (not republished works).

Please select one

Hardcover Book_____ or **Softcover Book**_____
Please select one

Editor/Author Details

Full name, affiliation and position:

Full contact address (including telephone and e-mail):

What is the approximate number of words and illustrations required for your proposed book (up to 200,000 words)? (Manuscripts consisting of 25,000-40,000 words are published in softcover only):

Words:_____ **Pages:**_____ **Illustrations:**_____ **Half/tones:**_____

Are color graphics necessary?_____

When will the complete manuscript be ready for submission? (Month/Year)

Projected Table of Contents:

Please state in detail the subject of the proposed publication and indicate its academic level:

Please include a 200-500 word descriptive paragraph which we could use for our website posting and brochures should a contract be signed:

Please give details of the principal audiences for the publication. List relevant subject areas and job functions.

What competitive publications are available?

What particular advantages does your publication have compared to the competitive publications?

How quickly do you think your publication might become out of date?

My recent Publications (past 5 years):

Figure/Template 4-16. Book Idea Proposal to Publisher.

INDEX